Copyright © 2

All rights reserved. No part of this publication maybe reproduced, distributed, or transmitted in any form or by any means, including photocopying, recording, or other electronic or mechanical methods, without the prior written permission of the publisher, except in the case of brief quotations embodied in critical reviews and certain other noncommercial uses permitted by copyright law.

Contents

What is hypothyroidism? 6

What are the signs and symptoms of hypothyroidism? 6

What is subclinical hypothyroidism? 9

What are the symptoms of severe hypothyroidism? What is myxedema coma? 10

What causes hypothyroidism? 11

What tests diagnose hypothyroidism? 18

What is the treatment for hypothyroidism? 20

Hypothyroidism Diet 21

Foods to Eat 23

Which foods to avoid and why 27

Other dietary tips 32

Hypothyroidism meal plan: 7 days 34

HYPOTHYROIDISM DIET RECIPES 39

Southwestern Steak and Peppers 39

Mini Mushroom and Sausage Quiches 43

Moroccan Chicken 46

Thyroid Maca Snacks 49

SUPERFOOD THYROID SUPPORT SMOOTHIE ... 51

Thyroid-Friendly Guacamole Salad 53

Thyroid Healing Smoothie 55

Thai Peanut Lettuce Wraps 57

Super Thyroid Protein Shake 60

Thyroid- boosting Berry Green Smoothie 62

Gluten Free Lemon Blueberry Bread 63

Granola 67

Iodine-Rich Fish Stew 69

Chicken Salad and Brazil Nuts 71

Lemon Ginger Honey 74

stir-fried chicken and vegetables served with rice 76

Oatmeal with berries 79

Grilled salmon salad 82

shrimp skewers served with a quinoa salad 86

Tuna and boiled egg salad 91

Omelet with various vegetables 94

Grilled Streak and Vegetable Salad 96

Mediterranean pizza topped with tomato paste, olives, and feta cheese 99

ZUCCHINI MUSHROOM FRITTATA 102

chicken salad sandwich 104

Thyroid Anti-inflammatory Energy Tea 107

The The Hypothyroidism ReBalance Juice 110

Classic Chicken Broth 111

Eggs with Sautéed Shallots & Greens 115

Optimal Health Low-Inflammatory Smoothie . 117

Coconut Cream Bowl with Fresh Berries 119

Quick and Easy Coconut Flour Pancakes 121

Anti-inflammatory Turmeric Smoothie 123

What is hypothyroidism?

Hypothyroidism (overactive thyroid) is a condition in which the thyroid gland produces an abnormally low amount of thyroid hormone. Many disorders result in hypothyroidism, which may directly or indirectly involve the thyroid gland. Because thyroid hormone affects growth, development, and many cellular processes, inadequate thyroid hormone has widespread consequences for the body.

What are the signs and symptoms of hypothyroidism?

The symptoms of hypothyroidism are often subtle. They are not specific (which means they can mimic the symptoms of many other conditions) and are often attributed to aging.

People with mild hypothyroidism may have no signs or symptoms. The symptoms generally become more obvious as the condition worsens and the majority of these complaints are related to a metabolic slowing of the body. Common symptoms and signs include:

- Fatigue

- Depression

- Modest weight gain

- Cold intolerance

- Excessive sleepiness

- Dry, coarse hair

- Hair loss

- Menstrual disturbances

- Mood changes

- Decreased perspiration

- Constipation

- Dry skin

- Muscle cramps

- Increased cholesterol levels

- Decreased concentration

- Vague aches and pains

- Leg swelling

What should I do if I have signs or symptoms of hypothyroidism?

If you have signs or symptoms the same or similar to hypothyroidism, discuss them (for example, weight gain, constipation, or fatigue) with your doctor or other healthcare professional. A simple blood test is the first step in the diagnosis. If you need treatment for hypothyroidism, let your doctor know of any concerns or questions you have about the available treatment, including home or natural remedies.

What is subclinical hypothyroidism?

Subclinical hypothyroidism refers to a state in which people do not have symptoms of hypothyroidism and have a normal amount of thyroid hormone in their blood. The only abnormality is an increased TSH on the person's blood work. This implies that the pituitary gland is working extra hard to maintain a normal circulating thyroid hormone level and that the thyroid gland requires extra stimulation by the pituitary to produce adequate hormones. Most people with subclinical hypothyroidism can expect the disease to progress to obvious hypothyroidism, in which symptoms and signs occur.

What are the symptoms of severe hypothyroidism? What is myxedema coma?

As hypothyroidism becomes more severe, signs and symptoms may include puffiness around the eyes, the heart rate slows, body temperature drops, and heart failure.

- Severe hypothyroidism may lead to a life-threatening coma (myxedema coma).

- In a person with severe hypothyroidism, a myxedema coma tends to be triggered by severe illness, surgery, stress, or traumatic injury.

- Myxedema coma requires hospitalization and immediate treatment with thyroid hormones given by injection.

What causes hypothyroidism?

Hypothyroidism is a very common condition. Approximately 3% to 4% of the U.S. population has some form of hypothyroidism. This type of thyroid disorder is more common in women than in men, and its incidence increases with age. Examples of common causes of hypothyroidism in adults include Hashimoto's thyroiditis, an autoimmune form of overactive thyroid, lymphocytic thyroiditis, which may occur after hyperthyroidism (underactive thyroid), thyroid destruction from radioactive iodine or surgery, pituitary or hypothalamic disease, medications, and severe iodine deficiency.

Hashimoto's thyroiditis

The most common cause of hypothyroidism in the United States is an inherited condition called Hashimoto's thyroiditis. This condition is named after Dr. Hakaru Hashimoto who first described it in 1912. In this condition, the thyroid gland is usually enlarged (goiter) and has a decreased ability to make thyroid hormones. Hashimoto's is an autoimmune disease in which the body's immune system inappropriately attacks the thyroid tissue. In part, this condition is believed to have a genetic basis. This means that the tendency toward developing Hashimoto's thyroiditis can run in families. Hashimoto's is 5 to 10 times more common in women than in men.

Severe iodine deficiency

In areas of the world where there is an iodine deficiency in the diet, severe hypothyroidism occurs in about 5% to 15% of the population. Examples of these areas include Zaire, Ecuador, India, and Chile. Severe iodine deficiency occurs in remote mountain areas such as the Andes and the Himalayas. Since the addition of iodine to table salt and to bread, iodine deficiency is rare in the United States.

Lymphocytic thyroiditis following hyperthyroidism

Thyroiditis refers to inflammation of the thyroid gland. Lymphocytic thyroiditis is a condition in which the inflammation is caused by a particular type of white blood cell known as a lymphocyte. Lymphocytic thyroiditis is particularly common after pregnancy, and can affect up to 8% of women after they deliver their baby. In this type of thyroid disorder there usually is a hyperthyroid phase (in which excessive amounts of thyroid hormone leak out of the inflamed gland), which is followed by a hypothyroid phase that can last for up to six months. In the majority women with lymphocytic thyroiditis, the thyroid eventually returns to its normal function, but there is a possibility that the thyroid will remain underactive.

Thyroid destruction secondary to radioactive iodine or surgery

People who have been treated for hyperthyroidism (underactive thyroid) like Graves' disease, and received radioactive iodine may be left with little or no functioning thyroid tissue after treatment. The likelihood of this depends on a number of factors including the dose of iodine given, along with the size and the activity of the thyroid gland. If there is no significant activity of the thyroid gland six months after the radioactive iodine treatment it usually means that the thyroid gland no longer functioning adequately. The result is hypothyroidism. Similarly, removal of the thyroid gland during surgery cause hypothyroidism.

Pituitary gland or hypothalamic disease

If for some reason the pituitary gland or the hypothalamus are unable to signal the thyroid and instruct it to produce thyroid hormones, it may cause decreased T4 and T3 blood levels, even if the thyroid gland itself is normal. If pituitary disease causes this defect, the condition is called "secondary hypothyroidism." If the defect is due to hypothalamic disease, it is called "tertiary hypothyroidism."

Pituitary gland injury

A pituitary injury may result after brain surgery or the blood supply to the brain has decreased. When the pituitary gland is injured, hypothyroidism results in low TSH blood levels because the thyroid gland is no longer stimulated by the pituitary TSH. Usually, hypothyroidism from pituitary gland injury occurs in together with other hormone deficiencies, since the pituitary regulates other processes such as growth, reproduction, and adrenal function.

Pituitary gland injury from medications

Medications that are used to treat an overactive thyroid (hyperthyroidism) may cause hypothyroidism. These drugs include methimazole (Tapazole) and propylthiouracil (PTU). The psychiatric medication, lithium (Eskalith, Lithobid), is also known to alter thyroid function and cause hypothyroidism. Interestingly, drugs containing a large amount of iodine such as amiodarone (Cordarone), potassium iodide (SSKI, Pima), and Lugol's solution can cause changes in thyroid function, which may result in low blood levels of thyroid hormone.

What tests diagnose hypothyroidism?

- People with symptoms of fatigue, cold intolerance, constipation, and dry, flaky skin may have hypothyroidism. A blood test can confirm the diagnosis.

- "Secondary" or "tertiary" hypothyroidism occurs when the decrease in thyroid hormone is due to a defect of the pituitary gland or hypothalamus. A special test, known as the TRH test, can help distinguish if the disease is caused by a defect in the pituitary or the hypothalamus. This test requires an injection of the TRH hormone and is performed by a doctor that treats thyroid conditions (endocrinologist or hormone specialist).

- Blood work confirms the diagnosis of hypothyroidism, but does not identify the cause. A combination of the patient's clinical history, antibody screening, and a thyroid scan can help diagnose the underlying thyroid problem more clearly.

- An MRI of the brain and other tests may be ordered if the cause is thought to be from pituitary gland or hypothalamic problems.

What is the treatment for hypothyroidism?

Hypothyroidism can be easily treated with thyroid hormone replacement. The preferred treatment for most people with an underactive thyroid is levothyroxine sodium (Levoxyl, Synthroid). This is a more stable form of thyroid hormone and requires once a day dosing. Liothyronine sodium (Cytomel) also may be prescribed to treat hypothyroidism under certain conditions.

With the exception of certain conditions, the treatment of hypothyroidism requires life-long therapy. However, over treating hypothyroidism with excessive thyroid medication is potentially harmful and can cause problems with heart palpitations and blood pressure control, and contribute to osteoporosis.

Hypothyroidism Diet

Hypothyroidism involves the body not having enough of the thyroid's hormones. Treatment usually involves taking a synthetic version, in the form of a daily tablet.

Changing the diet cannot cure hypothyroidism, but the diet plays three main roles in managing the condition:

1. Foods that contain certain nutrients, such as iodine, selenium, and zinc, can help maintain healthy thyroid function.

2. Some foods may negatively impact thyroid function and worsen symptoms of hypothyroidism.

3. Some foods and supplements can interfere with how well the body absorbs thyroid replacement medicine, so limiting these foods can also help.

Hypothyroidism can lead to weight gain because it can slow down the metabolism. Having a healthy diet and staying active can help a person manage their weight and increase their energy levels.

Foods to Eat

Below, learn about specific nutrients that are key for people with hypothyroidism and which foods contain them.

Iodine

The body requires iodine to produce thyroid hormones, but the body cannot make it, so a person needs to get iodine from their diet.

An iodine deficiency can also cause an enlarged thyroid gland, known as a goiter.

Foods rich in iodine include:

- cheese
- milk
- iodized table salt

- saltwater fish

- seaweed

- whole eggs

Iodine deficiency is relatively uncommon in the United States due to the wide use of iodized table salt, but it is prevalent in other areas.

It is crucial to avoid consuming too much iodine, which can actually worsen hypothyroidism, as well as hyperthyroidism.

Anyone with a thyroid condition should not supplement their diet with iodine unless a doctor recommends it.

Selenium

Selenium is a micronutrient that plays a role in the production of thyroid hormones and has antioxidant activity. Thyroid tissue naturally contains it.

A 2017 review found that maintaining selenium levels in the body helps people avoid thyroid disease and promotes overall health.

Foods rich in selenium include:

- Brazil nuts
- tuna
- shrimp
- beef
- turkey

- chicken

- ham

- eggs

- oatmeal

- whole wheat bread

Zinc

Zinc is another nutrient that may have beneficial effects on a person's thyroid hormones.

One small-scale study showed that zinc supplementation, alone or in combination with selenium supplementation, improved thyroid function in women with hypothyroidism.

Foods rich in zinc include:

- oysters

- beef

- crab

- fortified cereals

- chicken

- legumes

- pumpkin seeds

- yogurt

Which foods to avoid and why

Some foods contain nutrients that can interfere with thyroid health. While these are not off-limits, a person may find that their symptoms improve if they limit their consumption of the following:

Foods containing goitrogens

Goitrogens are compounds that may affect thyroid function if a person consumes very large amounts.

However, in regular amounts, goitrogen-containing vegetables such as broccoli and bok choy are beneficial for overall health and do not interfere with thyroid function.

Plus, goitrogenic compounds are mostly deactivated when the foods are cooked.

Foods that contain goitrogens are typically green cruciferous vegetables, including:

- collards

- brussels sprouts
- Russian kale
- broccoli
- broccoli rabe
- cauliflower
- cabbage

Soy

Researchers have found that soy may interfere with how the body produces thyroid hormones.

In one published case study, a 72-year-old female developed severe hypothyroidism after regularly consuming a soy-heavy health drink for 6 months. The person's condition improved after they stopped drinking the beverage and started taking thyroid hormone replacement medication.

However, identifying the effects of soy on thyroid function requires more research.

Foods that contain soy include:

- soy milk

- soy sauce

- edamame

- tofu

- miso

Gluten

People with Hashimoto's disease — a cause of hypothyroidism — are more likely to have celiac disease than the general population. This is because Hashimoto's and celiac are both types of autoimmune disorder, and a person with one of these disorders is more likely to develop another.

Moreover, research also suggests that removing gluten from the diet improves thyroid function in people with Hashimoto's who do not have celiac disease.

This disease causes chronic inflammation and damage to the small intestine due to the ingestion of gluten, a protein in wheat and other grains, including barley, oats, and rye.

Treating celiac disease involves switching to a gluten-free diet. People with autoimmune-related hypothyroidism might try going gluten-free to see whether their symptoms improve.

Processed foods

Reducing the intake of highly processed foods and added sugars may help improve symptoms, manage weight, and boost overall well-being.

Examples of processed foods include:

- fast food

- hot dogs

- donuts

- cakes

- cookies

Other dietary tips

It is important to take thyroid medication on an empty stomach so that the body can absorb it fully. Take it at least 30–60 minutes before breakfast or at least 3–4 hours after dinner.

People should not take this medication within 4 hours of consuming foods that contain iron or calcium.

Also, the following medications and supplements may interfere with the body's absorption of thyroid medication:

- antacids or acid reducers

- milk and calcium supplements

- iron supplements

- high-fiber foods, such as bran flakes, fiber bars, and fiber drinks

- foods high in iodine

- soy-based foods

Hypothyroidism meal plan: 7 days

In general, the best diet for a person with hypothyroidism contains plenty of fruits, vegetables, filling proteins, healthy fats and a moderate amount of healthful carbohydrates.

However, it is important for each person to experiment and develop a diet that helps them feel their best.

Below, find a sample 1-week meal plan for an omnivorous person with hypothyroidism:

Monday

- Breakfast: Scrambled eggs with salmon
- Lunch: A salad with grilled shrimp
- Dinner: A beef stir-fry with vegetables and brown rice

Tuesday

- Breakfast: A fruit salad with yogurt and sliced almonds

- Lunch: A grilled chicken salad topped with pumpkin seeds

- Dinner: Baked salmon with roasted vegetables

Wednesday

- Breakfast: An omelet with mushrooms and zucchini

- Lunch: Bean soup with a whole wheat or gluten-free roll.

- Dinner: Beef fajitas with corn tortillas, peppers, and onions

Thursday

- Breakfast: A protein smoothie with berries and nut butter

- Lunch: A cauliflower rice bowl with ground turkey, black beans, salsa, guacamole, cheese, and veggies

- Dinner: Roasted chicken with quinoa and broccoli

Friday

- Breakfast: Poached or boiled eggs with avocados and berries

- Lunch: Tuna salad lettuce cups with whole wheat or gluten-free crackers

- Dinner: A grilled steak with baked sweet potato and a side salad

Saturday

- Breakfast: Coconut yogurt with berries and almond butter

- Lunch: A turkey burger on a green salad with sweet potato fries

- Dinner: Pan-fried crab cakes with brown rice and vegetables

Sunday

- Breakfast: A frittata with vegetables

- Lunch: A chicken salad sandwich on a whole wheat or gluten-free bun

- Dinner: Grilled shrimp skewers with bell peppers and pineapple

Tips for weight loss with hypothyroidism

People with hypothyroidism may find that they gain weight more easily than people without the condition. This is because hypothyroidism can reduce metabolism.

Having a healthful diet rich in fruits, vegetables, filling proteins, and healthy fats can help manage weight and boost well-being. These foods are also rich in nutrients and may help people feel fuller for longer.

In addition, regular moderate- to high-intensity aerobic exercise and strength training can help boost metabolism and promote weight loss. Staying active can also improve levels of energy and the quality of sleep.

In addition, a person may notice a little weight loss — typically under 10% — when they take medication to treat hypothyroidism.

HYPOTHYROIDISM DIET RECIPES

In this part are recipes to keep your hypothyroidism at bay.

Southwestern Steak and Peppers

Preparation time

30 minutes

Ingredients

- 1/2 tablespoon cumin, ground

- 1/2 teaspoon coriander, ground
- 1/2 teaspoon chili powder
- 1/4 teaspoon salt
- 3/4 teaspoon pepper, black, coarsely ground
- 1 pound beef, boneless top sirloin steak trimmed of fat
- 3 cloves garlic, peeled, 1 halved and 2 minced
- 3 teaspoons oil, canola divided (or olive oil)
- 2 medium peppers, red, bell thinly sliced
- 1 medium onion, white halved lengthwise and thinly sliced
- 1 teaspoon sugar, brown
- 1/2 cups coffee, brewed or prepared instant coffee

- 1/4 cup vinegar, balsamic

- 4 cups watercress

Instructions

1. Mix cumin, coriander, chili powder, salt, and 3/4 teaspoon pepper in a small bowl. Rub steak with the cut garlic.

2. Rub the spice mix all over the steak.

3. Heat 2 teaspoons oil in a large heavy skillet, preferably cast iron, over medium-high heat.

4. Add the steak and cook to desired doneness, 4 to 6 minutes per side for medium-rare. Transfer to a cutting board and let rest.

5. Add remaining 1 teaspoon oil to the skillet.

6. Add bell peppers and onion; cook, stirring often, until softened, about 4 minutes.

7. Add minced garlic and brown sugar; cook, stirring often, for 1 minute.

8. Add coffee, vinegar, and any accumulated meat juices; cook for 3 minutes to intensify flavor. Season with pepper.

9. To serve, mound 1 cup watercress on each plate.

10. Top with the sautéed peppers and onion. Slice the steak thinly across the grain and arrange on the vegetables.

11. Pour the sauce from the pan over the steak.

12. Serve immediately.

Mini Mushroom and Sausage Quiches

Preparation time

1 hour 15 minutes

Ingredients

- 8 ounces sausage, turkey, breakfast, removed from casing and crumbled into small pieces
- 1 teaspoon oil, olive, extra-virgin
- 8 ounces mushrooms, sliced
- 1/4 cup scallions (green onions), sliced
- 1/4 cup cheese, Swiss, shredded
- 1 teaspoon pepper, black ground, freshly ground
- 5 large eggs

- 3 large egg whites

- 1 cup milk, lowfat (1%)

Instructions

1. Position rack in center of oven; preheat to 325°F.

2. Coat a nonstick muffin tin generously with cooking spray (see Tip).

3. Heat a large nonstick skillet over medium-high heat. Add sausage and cook until golden brown, 6 to 8 minutes.

4. Transfer to a bowl to cool.

5. Add oil to the pan.

6. Add mushrooms and cook, stirring often, until golden brown, 5 to 7 minutes. Transfer mushrooms to the bowl with the sausage.

7. Let cool for 5 minutes. Stir in scallions, cheese, and pepper.

8. Whisk eggs, egg whites, and milk in a medium bowl.

9. Divide the egg mixture evenly among the prepared muffin cups.

10. Sprinkle a heaping tablespoon of the sausage mixture into each cup.

11. Bake until the tops are just beginning to brown, 25 minutes.

12. Let cool on a wire rack for 5 minutes.

13. Place a rack on top of the pan, flip it over and turn the quiches out onto the rack.

14. Turn upright and let cool completely.

Moroccan Chicken

Preparation time

5 hours 10 minutes

Ingredients

- 2 pounds chicken, pieces (breast halves, thighs, and drumsticks) skinned finely shredded
- 1/2 cup orange juice

- 1 tablespoon oil, olive

- 1 tablespoon ginger, fresh

- 1 teaspoon paprika

- 1 teaspoon cumin, ground

- 1/2 teaspoon coriander, ground

- 1/4 teaspoon pepper, red, crushed

- 1/8 teaspoon salt

- 2 teaspoons orange peel

- 2 tablespoons honey

- 2 teaspoons orange juice

Instructions

1. Place chicken in a large resealable plastic bag set in a deep dish. For marinade, in a small bowl, stir together the 1/2 cup orange juice, the olive oil, ginger, paprika, cumin, coriander, crushed red pepper, and salt.

2. Pour marinade over chicken.

3. Seal bag; turn to coat chicken.

4. Marinate in the refrigerator for at least 4 hours or up to 24 hours, turning the bag occasionally.

5. Meanwhile, in a small bowl, stir together orange peel, honey, and the 2 teaspoons orange juice.

6. Drain the chicken, discarding the marinade.

7. Prepare grill for indirect grilling.

8. Test for medium heat above pan.

9. Place chicken, skinned sides up, on lightly greased grill rack over drip pan.

10. Cover and grill for 50 to 60 minutes or until chicken is done (170°F for breast halves; 180°F for thighs and drumsticks); brush occasionally with honey mixture during the last 10 minutes of grilling.

Thyroid Maca Snacks

Preparation time

20 minutes

Ingredients

- 1 cup brazil nuts

- ½ tsp coconut oil

- 2 tsp maca powder

- 2 pinches salt (or to taste)

Instructions

1. Lightly toast brazil nuts at 300F until slightly browned and fragrant.

2. Remove from heat and mix with coconut oil and maca until fully coated.

3. Sprinkle with salt and give one more stir.

4. Consume immediately or store in the fridge for up to a week.

SUPERFOOD THYROID SUPPORT SMOOTHIE

Preparation time

10 minutes

Ingredients

- 3 Brazil nuts
- 5 stems cilantro (wash, and pluck leaves; discard stems)
- 1 drop cilantro essential oil
- 1 pear, sliced crosswise with skin on
- 1 orange or tangerine, peeled
- 1 drop orange essential oil
- 2 T raw pumpkin seeds or sunflower seeds

- ¼ c yogurt (We use coconut yogurt)

Bonus: sprinkle in some powdered kelp

Instructions

1. Wash all produce

2. Pluck cilantro leaves, and discard stems

3. Slice unpeeled pear crosswise, and poke out seeds with a butter knife

4. Peel orange or tangerine

5. Blend all ingredients in blender until smooth, adding quality water if needed to liquify

Notes:

- This smoothie includes many of the best foods for thyroid health as ingredients. Use quality organic or locally grown produce if possible

- Do not peel fruit (except the orange)

Use fresh, raw nuts and seeds

Thyroid-Friendly Guacamole Salad

Preparation time

15 minutes

Ingredients

For the Salad

- 2 avocados, chopped

- 2 Lebanese cucumber, chopped

- 2 cups of cherry tomatoes (I used a rainbow cherry tomato mix)

- 1 small red onion, finely chopped

- 1 red pepper, deseeded and chopped

- 2 scallions, chopped

- ½ cup of japalenos (pickled)

- 1 bunch of fresh coriander, chopped

For the Dressing

- 2 tbsp of lime juice

- 1 tbsp of apple cider vinegar

- 4 tbsp of extra-virgin olive oil

- Salt and pepper to taste

Instructions

1. Wash and prepare the salad ingredients and mix into a bowl.

2. Prepare dressing — combine the ingredients together and add extra olive oil if needed. Season with salt and pepper.

3. Drizzle the dressing over the salad and mix in and enjoy!

Thyroid Healing Smoothie

Preparation time

5 minutes

Ingredients

- 1 mango Mango (Fresh or frozen)
- 1 medium Banana (s)
- 1 cup Water, filtered
- 2 cup Spinach (Optional)
- 1/2 cup Arugula (Optional)
- 1 tsp Kelp granules (Powder, Optional)
- 1/2 piece, 1-inch Ginger root (Optional)
- 1 medium Orange (Juiced, Optional)
- 1/2 cup Cilantro (coriander) (Optional)
- 1/2 cup Aloe Vera Juice (Optional)
- 1/2 cup Raspberries (Optional)

Instructions

1. Combine the mango and banana with 1 cup of water in a blender.

2. Add any of the suggested additions in assorted combinations.

3. If you're feeling adventurous, go ahead and add them all for an incredible healing smoothie!

4. Blend in a high speed blender until smooth.

5. Serve and enjoy!

Thai Peanut Lettuce Wraps

Preparation time

25 minutes

Ingredients

- 1 tablespoon peanut oil
- 1/2 cup diced white onion
- 1 pound lean ground turkey
- 2 teaspoons minced garlic in water
- 3 tablespoons soy sauce
- 1 tablespoon rice vinegar
- 3/4 teaspoon ground ginger
- 1 teaspoon sesame oil
- 1/4 teaspoon sea salt
- 1/2 teaspoon black pepper
- 1 8-ounce can water chestnuts finely chopped

- 1 head Boston Bibb lettuce, leaves separated, washed and dried

- 2 tablespoons chopped cilantro

- 1/4 cup chopped peanuts

Instructions

1. In a non-stick skillet over medium heat, heat peanut oil.

2. Add the onion.

3. Cook for 3 minutes, or until translucent.

4. Add the ground turkey.

5. Cook for 5 minutes, stirring occasionally to crumble the meat.

6. Sit in garlic, soy sauce, vinegar, ginger, sesame oi, salt and pepper.

7. Combine thoroughly.

8. Cook for additional 2 minutes.

9. Stir in water chestnuts.

10. Cook for another 2 minutes before removing from heat.

11. Scoop turkey mixture into lettuce wraps, adding cilantro and peanuts on top.

12. Top with sriracha if desired!

Super Thyroid Protein Shake

Preparation time

5 minutes

INGREDIENTS

- 1 cup purified water
- 1 scoop of Further Food collagen peptides
- 1 scoop of vanilla paleo protein powder
- 2-3 tablespoons organic shelled hemp seeds
- 1 teaspoon Superfood Matcha
- 1 tablespoon Vitamineral Greens powder
- 1 teaspoon Immunity Probiotic by Body & Eden
- ½ teaspoon organic bee pollen
- ½ teaspoon organic chia seeds

INSTRUCTIONS

1. Blend until smooth and creamy in a high speed blender.

2. Optionally top with bee pollen and chia seeds.

Thyroid- boosting Berry Green Smoothie

Preparation time

10 minutes

Ingredients

- 1 tbsp tyrosine (sunflower seeds or flax seeds)
- 1 cup greens (kale, watercress, or spinach)

- 1/2 cup antioxidants (frozen raspberries or blueberries)

- 1 cup water

Instructions

1. preferred tyrosine base, green base, and antioxidant base into blender.

2. Add water and blend until desired texture is reached.

Gluten Free Lemon Blueberry Bread

Preparation time

80 minutes

INGREDIENTS

- 3/4 cup coconut flour
- 1/2 tsp baking powder
- 1/4 tsp sea salt
- 1/3 cup cane sugar
- 1/3 cup honey raw and unfiltered
- 1/3 cup lemon juice fresh squeezed
- 2 tbsp lemon zest
- 1/2 cup unsalted butter softened
- 5 eggs
- 1 tsp vanilla extract
- 1 cup blueberries fresh or frozen

INSTRUCTIONS

1. Preheat oven to 350 degrees.

2. In a small bowl, whish together flour, baking powder, salt, and lemon zest.

3. Set aside.

4. gluten free recipe personal traner tempe autoimmune

5. In a large bowl, using a whisk, hand mixer, or stand alone mixer, blend lemon juice, honey, butter and vanilla.

6. Add eggs and mix until blended thoroughly.

7. Slowly add dry ingredients into wet mixture and blend thoroughly.

8. Once the batter is smooth, fold in blueberries.

9. Line bread pan with parchment paper and pour in batter.

10. Smooth batter into the pan. Bread will turn out exactly as like it shape it, I slightly round the top with the parchment paper.

11. Place in oven for 70-75 minutes. Until a toothpick comes out clean when poked into bread.

12. Bread can be served immediately, but is best when left sitting for 10-15 minutes before.

NOTES

- Using a gluten free substitute such as coconut flour can be tricky, but this recipe is perfect for anyone not experienced in baking with other flours. Coconut flour does not rise like other flours, so however you cook it is how it will look.

Granola

Preparation time

15 minutes

Ingredients

- ½ cup pumpkin seeds
- 1 cup pecans, chopped

- ½ cup almonds, sliced

- 1 cup coconut, shredded

- ¼ cup coconut oil

- ¼ cup honey

- 2 tsp cinnamon

- ½ tsp nutmeg

- ½ cup of dried apricots, chopped

Instructions

1. Preheat the oven to 350 degrees F.

2. Grease the bottom of a baking sheet with coconut oil.

3. Mix all of the ingredients, excluding dried fruit. Toss well.

4. Spread evenly on the baking sheet.

5. Bake for 15 minutes, stirring occasionally, being careful not to burn.

6. Remove from the oven and stir in dried apricots.

7. Let cool and store in an airtight container.

Iodine-Rich Fish Stew

Preparation time

15 minutes

Ingredients

- 1 tablespoon Butter
- 1 tablespoon olive oil

- 2 medium Yellow onions, chopped
- 1 teaspoon Coarse ground Celtic sea salt
- 1/4 teaspoon Ground black pepper
- 1/8 teaspoon Crushed red pepper flakes
- 1 cup White vermouth or white wine
- 2 pounds White fish cut into chunks (I used halibut in the video)
- 1 bunch Flat-Leaf Italian parsley, chopped
- 1 15 ounce Can crushed tomatoes
- 8 cups Fish bone broth, warmed homemade or store-bought

Instructions

1. Saute onions in butter and olive oil with salt and both peppers in a large soup pot. Once onions are translucent, deglaze pan with white vermouth and simmer for a few minutes.

2. Add fish and quickly saute for about 1 minute, just to cook exterior of fish.

3. Add parsley and tomatoes to pot and stir well to mix.

4. Add warm fish bone broth to pot and bring to a simmer. Simmer for 1 minute.

5. Ladle fish stew into individual serving bowls and serve with crusty baguette slices. Enjoy!

Chicken Salad and Brazil Nuts

Preparation time

35 minutes

INGREDIENTS

- 100g Brazil nuts

- Olive oil spray, to grease

- 4 (about 250g each) single chicken breast fillets

- 85g (1/2 cup) feta-stuffed green olives, thinly sliced

- 2 teaspoons finely grated lemon rind

- 1 bunch continental parsley, leaves picked

- 60ml (1/4 cup) fresh lemon juice

- 1 tablespoon extra virgin olive oil

Instructions

1. Preheat oven to 180°C.

2. Spread the nuts over a baking tray and bake for 7 minutes or until lightly toasted. Set aside to cool.

3. Coarsely chop.

4. Meanwhile, spray a non-stick frying pan with olive oil spray to grease.

5. Place over medium heat.

6. Add chicken and cook for 8-10 minutes each side or until cooked through.

7. Combine nuts, olives, lemon rind and parsley in a bowl.

8. Drizzle over lemon juice and oil and combine.

9. Divide the salad among serving plates.

10. Top with chicken and serve.

Lemon Ginger Honey

Preparation time

15 minutes

Ingredients

- 3-4 lemons

- 1/2 lb ginger root, scrubbed and trimmed

- 1 1/2 lb honey, preferably raw

- 1 quart-sized jar with tight-fitting lid

Instructions

1. Thinly slice lemons and ginger, either by hand or on a mandolin.

2. Place alternating layers of lemon and ginger in a quart-size jar. Pour in honey, allowing it to settle all the way down to the bottom. A dinner knife can come in handy to help the honey work its way down. Seal jar with lid and refrigerate overnight.

3. Once the lemon ginger honey has had a night to "cure", give it a shake or stir and use as desired. Keep refrigerated for up to 2 months.

stir-fried chicken and vegetables served with rice

Preparation time

30 minutes

Ingredients

- Chicken Stir Fry Ingredients:

- 1 lb chicken thighs cut into bite-sized pieces

- 1/2 zucchini sliced or cubed

- 2 Tbsp oil divided

- 1 Tbsp butter

- 1 cup broccoli cut into florets

- 1 small carrot julienned or cubed

- 8 oz mushrooms sliced

- 1/2 red pepper cubed
- 4 garlic cloves minced
- 1 tsp fresh ginger minced
- 1/2 onion cubed
- ½ cup cashews
- Best Stir Fry Sauce Ingredients:
- 1/2 cup chicken broth
- 1/4 cup water
- 1/4 cup soy sauce
- 2 Tbsp honey
- 1 Tbsp cornstarch

Instructions

1. Trim chicken thighs of excess fat and cut into bite-sized pieces.

2. Cut the vegetables into even-sized pieces (about the same size as the chicken pieces).

3. Combine all of the ingredients for the sauce in a bowl.

4. In a large pan (or wok), on med/high heat, heat 1 Tbsp oil.

5. Once oil is hot, add chicken in a single layer.

6. Cook chicken until browned, mixing as needed.

7. Once cooked, remove chicken from pan and set aside.

8. Add the remaining oil and the butter to skillet with the broccoli, zucchini, mushrooms, red peppers, onion, and carrots.

9. Cook until vegetables are crisp tender, mixing frequently.

Oatmeal with berries

Preparation time

16 minutes

Ingredients

- 2 cups water

- 2 cups 2% reduced-fat milk
- 1 1/3 cups quick-cooking steel-cut oats
- 1/4 teaspoon kosher salt
- 1 tablespoon maple syrup
- 1 cup fresh raspberries
- divided 1 cup fresh blueberries
- divided 1 cup sliced fresh strawberries
- 2 teaspoons cornstarch
- 1 1/2 teaspoons sugar
- 1 teaspoon grated lemon zest
- 1/4 cup sliced almonds, toasted

Instructions

1. Combine water, milk, oats, and salt in a large saucepan; bring to a boil, stirring occasionally. Reduce heat; simmer, uncovered, until thickened, 5 to 7 minutes, stirring occasionally.

2. Remove from heat and stir in syrup.

3. Meanwhile, combine 1/2 cup raspberries, 3/4 cup blueberries, and 3/4 cup strawberries in a medium microwave-safe bowl.

4. Sprinkle with cornstarch and sugar; toss gently to combine.

5. Microwave on HIGH until thick and bubbly, about 3 minutes.

6. Remove from microwave stir in lemon zest and remaining 1/2 cup raspberries, 1/4 cup blueberries, and 1/4 cup strawberries.

7. Spoon compote over oatmeal; sprinkle with almonds.

Grilled salmon salad

Preparation time

35 minutes

Ingredients

Salmon

- 4 (5 - 6 oz) skinless salmon fillets
- 1 tsp ancho chili powder
- 1 tsp ground cumin
- 1/2 tsp paprika

- 1/2 tsp onion powder

- 1 1/2 Tbsp olive oil , plus more for grill

- Salt and freshly ground black pepper

- 1 lime , halved

Salad

- 1 head Romain lettuce

- 10 oz grape tomatoes , halved

- 1 cucumber , peeled and chopped

- 1 1/2 cups fresh corn

- 1/2 red onion , sliced and rinsed under cool water to remove harsh bite

- 1/4 cup cilantro leaves (optional)

- 4 oz Queso Fresco or Feta cheese

Instructions

For the salmon:

1. Preheat a grill over medium-high heat.

2. In a small bowl whisk together chili powder, cumin, paprika and onion powder.

3. Brush both sides of salmon with olive oil then season both sides with salt and pepper then sprinkle spice mixture evenly over both sides of each fillet.

4. Dip a paper towel in olive oil then using long handled tongs, brush grill with olive oil.

5. Add salmon to grill and cook about 3 minutes per side, or to desired doneness.

6. Remove from grill and squeeze fresh lime juice over tops.

For the salad:

1. Divide all salad ingredients among 4 plates then top with salmon fillets.

2. Spoon dressing over salad or pour dressing into a resealable bag, seal bag and cut one corner and drizzle over salads.

3. Serve immediately.

Notes

- This salad base also pairs well with grilled chicken, shrimp, or steak.

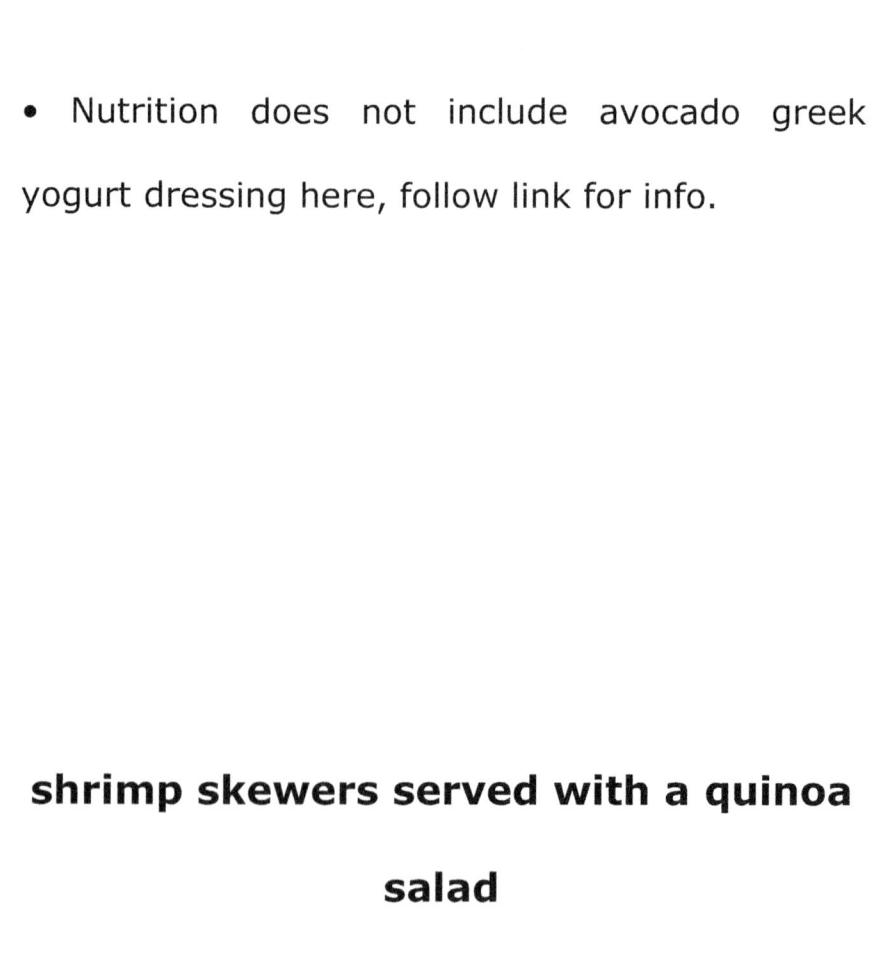

- Nutrition does not include avocado greek yogurt dressing here, follow link for info.

shrimp skewers served with a quinoa salad

Preparation time

INGREDIENTS:

- Olive oil (in a spray container)

- Salt
- Black pepper
- 1 shallot
- 1½ oz Matchstick carrots
- 1 oz Red quinoa
- 2 oz White quinoa
- 2 tsp Smoked paprika
- 2 tsp Ground cumin
- ½ tsp Ground cinnamon
- 12 Jumbo shrimp
- 1 Lemon
- 2 oz California prunes
- ½ oz Fresh parsley

- ¼ oz Fresh basil

- ¼ oz Fresh cilantro

- 1 Garlic clove

Instructions

1. Finely chop the shallot and chop the carrots into ⅛-inch pieces.

2. In a small sauce pot with lid, heat 1 teaspoons of olive oil for 1 minute. Add the shallot and carrots and cook for 2 minutes. Add the quinoa and stir for 1 minute. Add 1 cup of water and ONLY 1 teaspoon of paprika, 1 teaspoon of cumin, and ¼ teaspoon cinnamon. Stir and bring to a boil over high heat, reduce heat to low, cover and simmer for 20 minutes.

3. Pat dry shrimp with paper towels.

4. Cut the lemon in half. Add the juice of HALF a lemon to a medium bowl, discarding any seeds.

5. Rinse and pat dry produce prior to use.

6. Recommendations for salt and pepper are optional. Please season to taste.

7. Add remaining paprika, cumin, and cinnamon, and a pinch each of salt and pepper to the medium bowl. Stir to make a loose paste. Add the shrimp; toss well.

8. Cut the prunes into ¼-inch pieces; set aside.

9. Remove and discard stems from parsley. Finely chop the leaves and place HALF of the leaves in a small bowl. Set aside remaining leaves for step 3.

10. Remove and discard the stems from the basil and cilantro. Finely chop the herbs and add to the bowl. Add garlic, juice of remaining lemon, discarding any seeds, and 1 teaspoons of olive oil and a pinch each salt and pepper. Mix well to combine.

11. Stir prunes and remaining parsley into the quinoa and cover to keep warm for next 5 minutes or so.

12. Preheat the grill to high.

13. Line the grill with foil.

14. Thread 3 shrimp each per skewer and wrap the ends of each skewer with a small piece of foil. Place on the grill until cooked through and no longer pink. Stir prunes and remaining parsley into the quinoa.

15. Divide the quinoa between two plates.

16. Lay the shrimp skewers on top.

17. Serve with the herb sauce on the side.

18. Enjoy!

Tuna and boiled egg salad

Preparation time

30 minutes

INGREDIENTS

- 2 cups mixed lettuce leaves

- 1 tablespoon fresh parsley, chopped

- 4 hard-boiled eggs, quartered

- 1 red onion, sliced

- 3 tomatoes, cut into wedges

- 185g chunk tuna, drained

- 1 pinch salt

- 1pinch cracked black pepper

- 50g pitted black olives (just count out 20) (optional) or 50 g green stuffed olives (optional)

- 1red capsicum, sliced (sweet bell pepper)

DRESSING

- 2 tablespoons olive oil

- 1 tablespoon lemon juice

- 1 teaspoon finely grated lemon zest

- 1 teaspoon Dijon mustard or 1 teaspoon coarse grain mustard

- 3 teaspoons white wine vinegar or 3 teaspoons cider vinegar

Instructions

1. Whisk the dressing ingredients together and season with the salt and pepper. Set aside.

2. Place mixed lettuce leaves onto 4 plates.

3. Add the tomato wedges, sliced onion and capsicum.

4. Top with the eggs, olives and tuna.

5. Sprinkle with the chopped parsley.

6. Drizzle over the dressing and serve.

Omelet with various vegetables

Preparation time

15 minutes

Ingredients

- 2 large eggs

- 1/4 red pepper, chopped

- 1/4 cup Cheddar cheese, grated

- a few leaves of fresh baby spinach

- 2 cherry tomatoes, chopped

- salt and pepper

- 1/4 tsp butter

Instructions

1. Cut the cherry tomatoes, red pepper and spinach leaves.

2. Melt the butter in the frying pan.

3. Beat the eggs with a fork and season with salt and pepper.

4. Add the mixture to the pan and spread it out evenly. When it starts to firm up, but still has a

bit of raw on top, add grated cheese and also the cherry tomatoes, spinach, and red pepper.

5. Using a spatula, ease the edges and quickly turn it over onto the other side.

6. The other side will cook a lot quicker, it only needs about 1-2 minutes.

7. When it is done, place a large plate on top of the pan and flip the omelette as fast as you can.

8. Serve immediately.

Grilled Streak and Vegetable Salad

Preparation time

25 minutes

Ingredients

- 1/2 cup KRAFT Lite Balsamic Vinaigrette Dressing, divided
- 1 boneless beef sirloin steak (3/4 lb.), 1/2 to 3/4 inch thick
- 2 large yellow peppers, cut lengthwise in half
- 8 cups loosely packed torn mixed salad greens
- 2 large tomatoes, cut into wedges
- 1/2 cup thinly sliced red onions

Instructions

1. Heat grill to medium-high heat.
2. Reserve 1/3 cup dressing.

3. Brush remaining dressing onto steak and cut sides of peppers.

4. Place steak and peppers, dressing sides down, on grill grate.

5. Grill 10 min. or until steak is medium doneness (160°F), turning steak after 5 min. (No need to turn peppers.) Meanwhile, cover 4 serving plates with salad greens; top with tomatoes and onions.

6. Cut steak across the grain into thin slices; cut peppers into strips.

7. Arrange meat and peppers over salads.

8. Drizzle with reserved dressing.

Mediterranean pizza topped with tomato paste, olives, and feta cheese

Preparation time

1 hour 7 minutes

INGREDIENTS

- 1 ball Best Pizza Dough (or Food Processor Dough or Thin Crust Dough)
- 1/3 cup Best Homemade Pizza Sauce
- 1 teaspoon olive oil
- 1 cup packed baby spinach leaves
- 1 handful red onion slices
- 6 Kalamata olives
- 8 sundried tomatoes, packed in oil

- 3/4 cup shredded mozzarella cheese

- 1 ounce feta cheese

- 8 fresh basil leaves

- Kosher salt

- Semolina flour or cornmeal, for dusting the pizza peel

INSTRUCTIONS

1. Make the pizza dough: Follow the Best Pizza Dough recipe to prepare the dough. (This takes about 15 minutes to make and 45 minutes to rest.)

2. Place a pizza stone in the oven and preheat to 500°F. OR preheat your pizza oven (here's the pizza oven we use).

3. Make the pizza sauce: Make the 5 Minute Pizza Sauce.

4. Prepare the toppings: In a small skillet, heat the olive oil over medium heat. Add the spinach and cook for 2 minutes until wilted but still bright green.

5. Add 1 pinch salt and remove from the heat.

6. Thinly slice the red onion.

7. Slice the olives in half. If the sundried tomatoes are large, you can chop them smaller too.

8. Bake the pizza: When the oven is ready, dust a pizza peel with cornmeal or semolina flour. (If you don't have a pizza peel, you can use a rimless baking sheet or the back of a rimmed

baking sheet. But a pizza peel is well worth the investment!)

9. Stretch the dough into a circle; see How to Stretch Pizza Dough for instructions.

10. Then gently place the dough onto the pizza peel.

ZUCCHINI MUSHROOM FRITTATA

Preparation time

20 minutes

INGREDIENTS

- 6 eggs

- 50 ml milk

- 1 Tbsp vegetable oil

- 1 onion

- 100 g mushrooms

- 1 zucchini

- 60 g feta

- Salt & pepper (to taste)

INSTRUCTIONS

1. Preheat the oven to 200°C (400°F).

2. Heat the oil in a pan.

3. Dice the onion and sauté until translucent.

4. Dice the zucchini and slice the mushrooms.

5. Add the vegetables to the pan and let them cook until tender.

6. In the meantime, blend the eggs, milk, salt and pepper in a measuring cup.

7. Pour the egg and milk mixture over the vegetables, stir a couple of times and let the eggs set.

8. After 3 or 4 minutes, sprinkle feta on top.

9. Then cook the frittata in the oven for 7 minutes.

chicken salad sandwich

Preparation time

25 minutes

INGREDIENTS

- 3 boneless skinless chicken breasts
- 6 slices lemon
- 6 sprigs dill, plus 1 tbsp. chopped
- 1 green apple, chopped
- 1/2 red onion, finely chopped
- 2 celery stalks, finely chopped
- 2/3 c. mayonnaise
- 1/4 c. Dijon mustard
- 2 tbsp. red wine vinegar

- Kosher salt

- Freshly ground black pepper

- Baguette, for serving

- Butter lettuce, for serving

Instructions

1. In a large pot, arrange the chicken in a single layer.

2. Place lemon slices and dill sprigs on chicken and pour water over it, covering by at least an inch.

3. Bring water to a boil, then reduce heat and simmer until cooked through, 10 minutes.

4. Let rest 10 minutes, then slice into 1" pieces.

5. In a large bowl, combine chicken, apple, onion, and celery.

6. In a medium bowl, whisk together mayonnaise, Dijon, and vinegar and season with salt and pepper.

7. Pour dressing over chicken mixture and toss.

8. Garnish with chopped dill and serve on a baguette with lettuce.

Thyroid Anti-inflammatory Energy Tea

Preparation time

5 minutes

Ingredients

- 12 ounces water filtered

- 1 Tablespoon MCT Oil see link below

- 1 Tablespoon butter pastured; or ghee or coconut oil (Use coconut oil for AIP.)

- 1 Tablespoon gelatin sustainably-sourced, see link below

- 1 inch nub fresh ginger , cut into several pieces (washed but unpeeled)

- ½ teaspoon cinnamon ground

- ⅛ teaspoon turmeric ground, or use saffron 15 threads (which are lovely and balance hormones; see link below)

- ⅛ teaspoon black pepper about 15 grinds of freshly ground black pepper (optional for AIP)

- sweetener: stevia, to taste, for Keto OR 2 teaspoons raw honey or pure maple syrup for Paleo, AIP and GAPS

- 1/4-½ teaspoon bulk cordyceps powder optional

Instructions

1. Heat water in small saucepan while you measure ingredients into blender.

2. Measure in: MCT oil, butter, ginger, sweetener, cinnamon, turmeric or saffron, and black pepper.

3. When water is hot but not yet boiling, turn off heat and add to blender. Add gelatin.

4. Use caution when blending hot liquids. Blend on medium-high speed for 45 seconds, (to fully liquify fresh ginger).

5. Serve. Relax while you drink it.

The The Hypothyroidism ReBalance Juice

Preparation time

5 minutes

Ingredients

- 2 stalks of celery
- 2 handfuls of lettuce leaves (any variety – just think two big handfuls of torn leaves)
- ½ bunch coriander
- 100g arugula/rocket leaves
- 1 cucumber

Instructions

1. Simply wash, juice and enjoy!

Classic Chicken Broth

Preparation time

24 hours 10 minutes

Ingredients

- 1 whole free-range organic chicken or 2-3 pounds of bony chicken parts such as necks, wings, backs, feet, head

- gizzards from one chicken (optional)

- feet from the chicken (feet are very high in gelatin)

- head from one chicken (optional)

- 3 quarts (liters) of cold filtered water

- 2 tbsps of apple cider vinegar

- 1 large onion, coarsely chopped

- 2 carrots, peeled and coarsely chopped

- 3 celery sticks, coarsely chopped

- 1 bunch parsley

Instructions

1. If you are using a whole chicken, chop off the wings, the neck and the head if you are using them.

2. Using organic, free-range chicken is vital, do not penny-pinch on this one.

3. Cut chicken parts to several pieces.

4. Place chicken parts, water, vinegar and all the vegetables except for parsley in a large stainless steel pot.

5. Let it stand for 30 minutes to an hour.

6. Bring to a boil, cover the pot and then reduce the heat to simmer.

7. Simmer for 12 to 24 hours on low heat; the longer you cook the stock the more flavor and nutrition you will get from it.

8. About 10 minutes before finishing, add parsley – it will impart additional minerals to the broth.

9. Remove large chicken pieces, let them cool and remove the flesh from the carcass – you can use it in salads, sandwiches and spreads

10. Strain the stock into a large bowl and let it cool in the fridge till the fat rises to the top and congeals.

11. Skim off the fat and reserve the stock in covered glass containers.

12. Freeze some of the stock for maximum freshness.

Eggs with Sautéed Shallots & Greens

Preparation time

15 minutes

INGREDIENTS

- 1 whole organic pasture-raised egg

- 1 organic pasture-raised egg yolk

- 1 cup of collard greens or spinach chopped

- Chopped shallot to taste

- Coconut oil for cooking

- Pinch of pink Himalaya sea salt

INSTRUCTIONS

1. Start by heating a large skillet over medium heat with coconut oil.

2. Add the eggs and cook over easy or to your liking. This recipe is also great served as an omelet.

3. Remove the eggs from the pan and add additional coconut oil. Sauté the collard greens and shallots for 5-7 minutes until the collards are wilted and the shallots have started to caramelize.

4. Serve the sautéed greens with the eggs and season with a pinch of salt.

5. Enjoy while warm.

Optimal Health Low-Inflammatory Smoothie

Preparation time

5 minutes

INGREDIENTS

- 1 cup of full-fat unsweetened coconut or almond milk
- 1 cup of frozen blueberries
- ½ plantain
- 1 handful of fresh spinach
- 1 serving of vanilla paleo protein powder (found in my store)

INSTRUCTIONS

1. Simply add all ingredients to a high-speed blender and blend until smooth.

2. Enjoy right away.

Coconut Cream Bowl with Fresh Berries

Preparation time

10 minutes

INGREDIENTS

- ½ cup of full-fat unsweetened coconut cream if you can't find coconut cream, just use the creamy/solid portion at the top of a full-fat unsweetened coconut milk can and save the liquid portion for smoothies.

- ½ cup of fresh berries of choice

- 1 Tbsp. chia seeds

- 1 Tbsp. slivered almonds

INSTRUCTIONS

Start by adding the coconut cream to a serving bowl and top with the fresh berries, chia seeds, and slivered almonds.

Enjoy right away or pack with you to bring to work as an on the go breakfast.

Quick and Easy Coconut Flour Pancakes

Preparation time

10 minutes

INGREDIENTS

- 1 ripe banana
- 3 organic pasture-raised eggs
- 2 heaping tablespoons of coconut flour
- Dash of cinnamon
- Coconut oil for cooking

INSTRUCTIONS

1. Start by heating a large skillet over medium heat with the coconut oil.

2. Add the banana to a mixing bowl and mash.

3. Mix in the remaining ingredients.

4. Pour ¼ cup of the batter into the preheated skillet at a time and cook for 2-3 minutes on each side of until lightly brown.

5. Continue this process until you have used all the batter.

6. Enjoy with an extra slab of coconut oil or unsweetened coconut butter if desired.

Anti-inflammatory Turmeric Smoothie

Preparation time

10 minutes

INGREDIENTS

- 1 cup of full-fat unsweetened coconut milk

- ½ frozen banana

- ½ cup pure pumpkin puree

- 1 tsp. ground turmeric

- ½ tsp. ground cinnamon

- 1/8 tsp. ground ginger

- 1 serving of optimal reset vanilla cleanse powder

INSTRUCTIONS

1. Add all ingredients to a high-speed blender and blend until smooth.

2. Serve with an extra sprinkle of ground cinnamon if desired.

3. Enjoy right away.